Unleashed
Transforming My Battle With Depression

Saundra Jain, MA, PsyD, LPC
& Rakesh Jain, MD, MPH

A Mental Aerobics Project

This book is dedicated to our patients –
the best of all teachers.

ACKNOWLEDGEMENTS

We offer thanks and appreciation to our friends and colleagues for reading the manuscript and offering insightful, thoughtful comments.

We express our deep and heartfelt gratitude to our parents. Their patience, encouragement, and never-ending faith are the foundation for our many successes. Last, but definitely not least, we thank our son, Nick, for his support and sharing in the fun.

INTRODUCTION

Today's world is fast paced and filled with opportunities and responsibilities. Depression and anxiety are headline news and are frequently featured on talk shows. We now have a better awareness and understanding of these problems thanks to televised and written media. People are beginning to talk about these problems and seek help.

We work in the field of mental health. Saundra is a psychotherapist and Rakesh is a psychiatrist. We are privileged to work with individuals and families struggling with depression and anxiety. A problem we deal with frequently is medication non-adherence.

People are often resistant to the idea of medication due to perceived stigma, fear of ridicule, and shame. People quit taking their medication for many reasons including side effects and lack of improvement. Others may stop taking their medication because they feel better but they are at risk of the symptoms returning.

We encounter these struggles on a daily basis. The patients' concerns and worries are varied and each deserves respect and consideration. We decided to write a book of affirmations for people dealing with the decision to take or continue taking medication for depression and anxiety. The book offers support and guidance when faced with this decision. This is an illness that affects entire family systems. Its impact far exceeds the boundaries of the family and reaches into the community, workplace, and social relationships.

The title, *UNLEASHED: Transforming My Battle with Depression*, was a gift from one of our patients. After hearing about the book and remembering her days of feeling shackled by depression, she smiled and said, "UNLEASHED.... once I began taking anti-depressants my life was transformed." As we noted in the acknowledgement, patients are our best teachers so take a moment and read how she describes her experiences with depression and anxiety.

*I felt in **bondage**.*

I didn't want to be in public. I would get so nervous. I felt like everyone could see how unhappy I was. I felt ugly and worthless. I knew that everyone else felt that way about me too.

The ones I loved the most didn't like being with me. I would complain and get angry when people didn't listen to my advice or suggestions. I would get sad. I wanted my family to make me feel better. They didn't know how. I didn't know how. They wanted to live life and enjoy it. I couldn't! I thought if they would stay around I would be happy. I pushed them away because they would get depressed being around me. They didn't want to sit in the house all the time. My marriage was in jeopardy. My children didn't feel they could confide in me. I felt like they were pushing me away but I was pushing my family away.

I felt like I was behind a brick wall. I wanted to crawl over but I didn't know how to get that far. Something kept me from getting up and climbing over that wall. I wanted to have fun. I wanted to be included. I wanted to laugh. I just couldn't. But when people tried to help, I got angry because they thought I was giving up. I wasn't giving up. I JUST COULDN'T DO IT. It was as though I was leashed on a chain, not able to stretch or go that far. People were giving up on me. I was giving up on myself.

I knew something had to change. When I saw commercials on TV about medicine helping people I thought, "Maybe for someone else but not for me." Thank goodness I was wrong. When I started taking medication it was as if someone handed me a key and I unlocked the chains that were holding me behind that brick wall - trapped in a world that most people never experience - a dark and cold world. Medication helped me crawl over that wall into a bright and beautiful world that is warm and wonderful. WITH MY FAMILY!! It is a totally different world!

Not everyone is so lucky. I try to share my experiences with others having the same problem. I tell them that medications are just like clothes – Not all of us can wear the same style and look good in them. We have to try something else. That's how it is with medicine. There is something out there for you. You just have to keep trying until you find the right one for you!

What an amazing story of strength and courage when confronted with these devastating disorders. This book offers positive affirmations to anyone confronted with the problem of depression and anxiety, especially when taking medication. We hope this book serves as a source of strength for anyone who reads it.

Turn the page and begin your journey! It is filled with the power of choice and words promoting strength and well being. Travel the pages with a sense of serenity and growth and find the key to unlock those chains!

Enjoy.....

Saundra & Rakesh

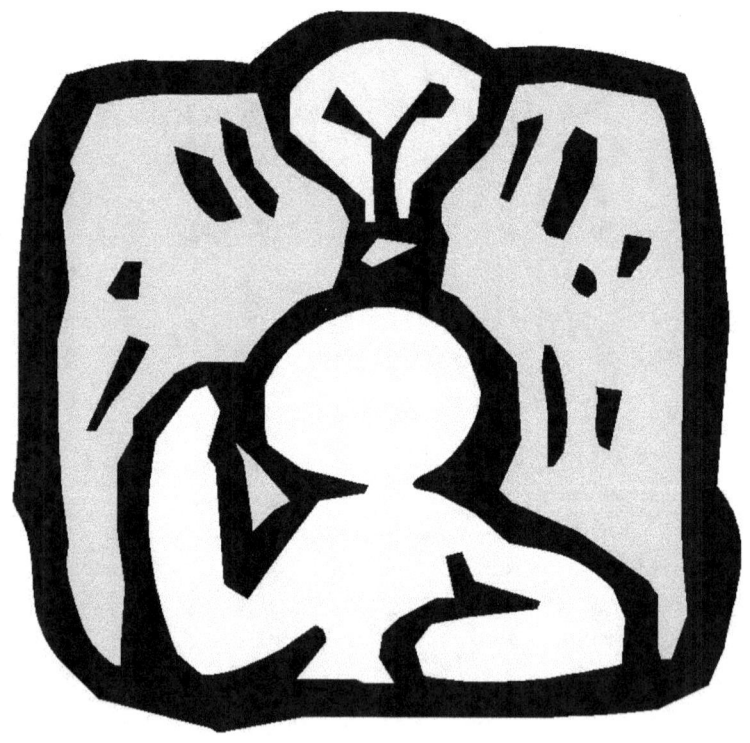

I recognize and accept the power of positive thought in my daily life. Positive thoughts counteract the negative thoughts associated with depression and anxiety. I will continuously train my mind to generate an abundance of positive thoughts. This I promise myself.

Reflections: _____

_____

_____

_____

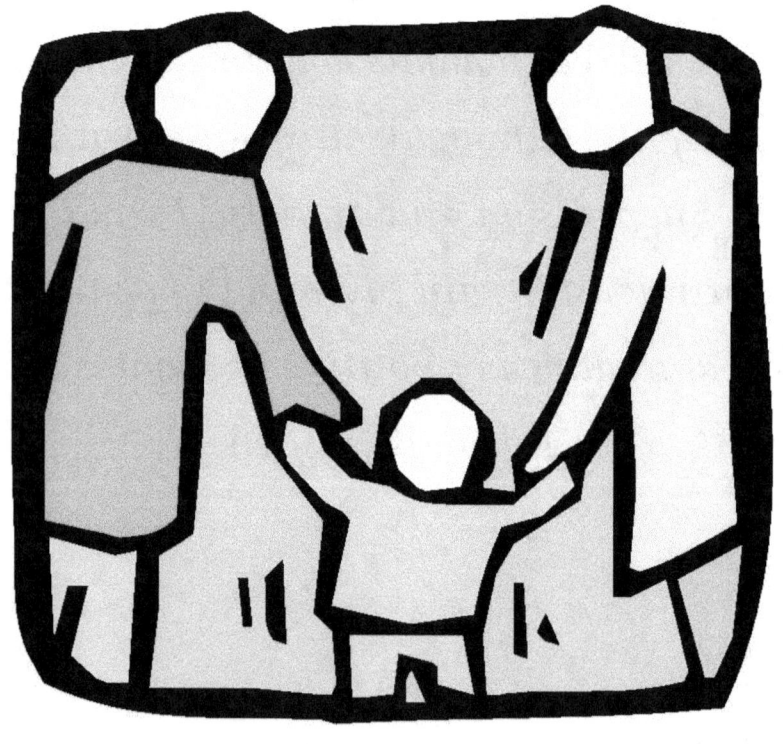

Medication assists me in dealing with depression and anxiety in a positive way. Medication enables me to deal with stress and day-to-day problems more effectively. Best of all, I am a better friend, spouse, and parent.

Reflections: _____

_____

_____

_____

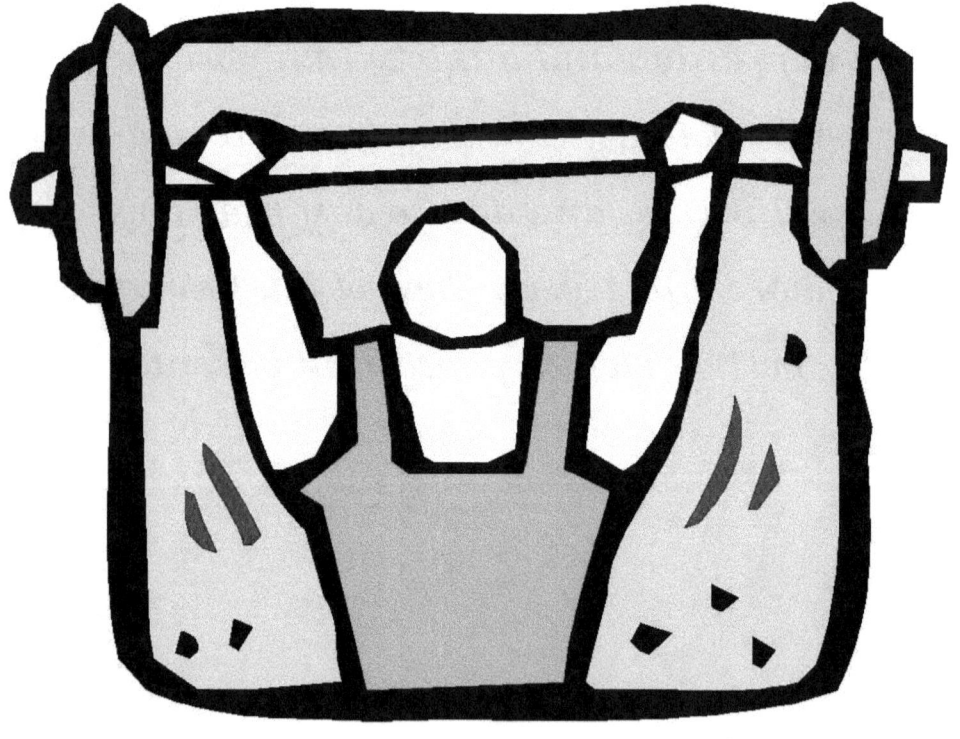

I promise to view taking medication as a sign of strength not weakness. It represents my commitment to health and a willingness to recognize a problem I can overcome.

Reflections: _____

_____

_____

_____

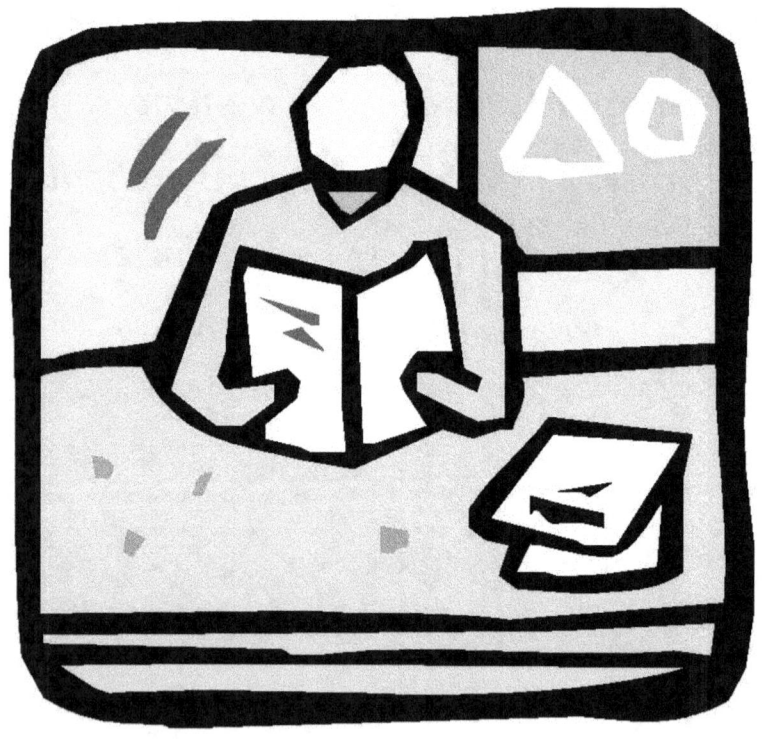

It is my choice to be on medication for depression and anxiety. I have educated myself about the illness of depression and anxiety and the available treatment options. I am empowered by the choices I make.

Reflections: _____

_____

_____

_____

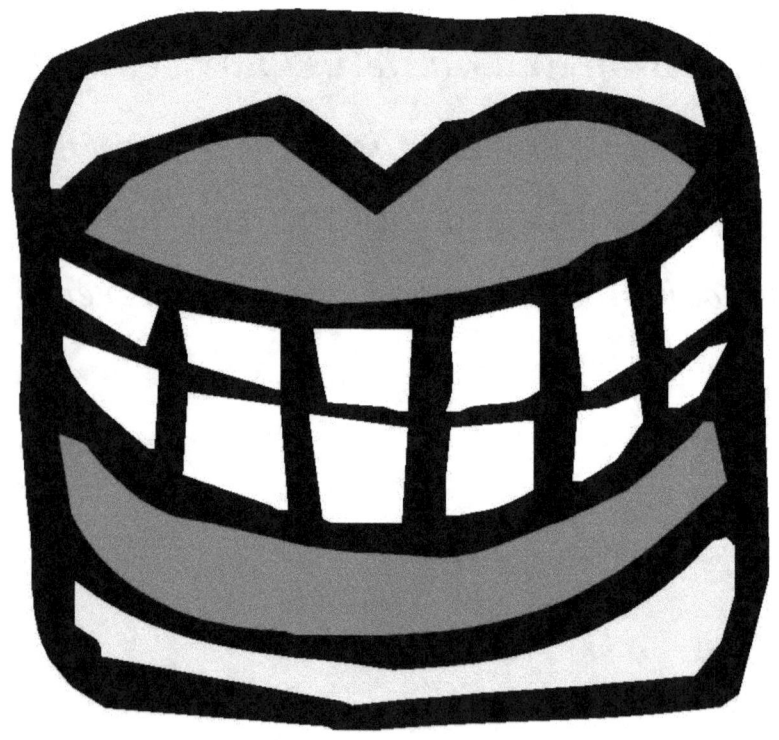

If others criticize my decision to take medication I will not take it personally. Their criticism will not hurt me nor steer me off course in my journey toward mental health. I promise to respond to their comments with tolerance and humor.

Reflections: _____

_____

_____

_____

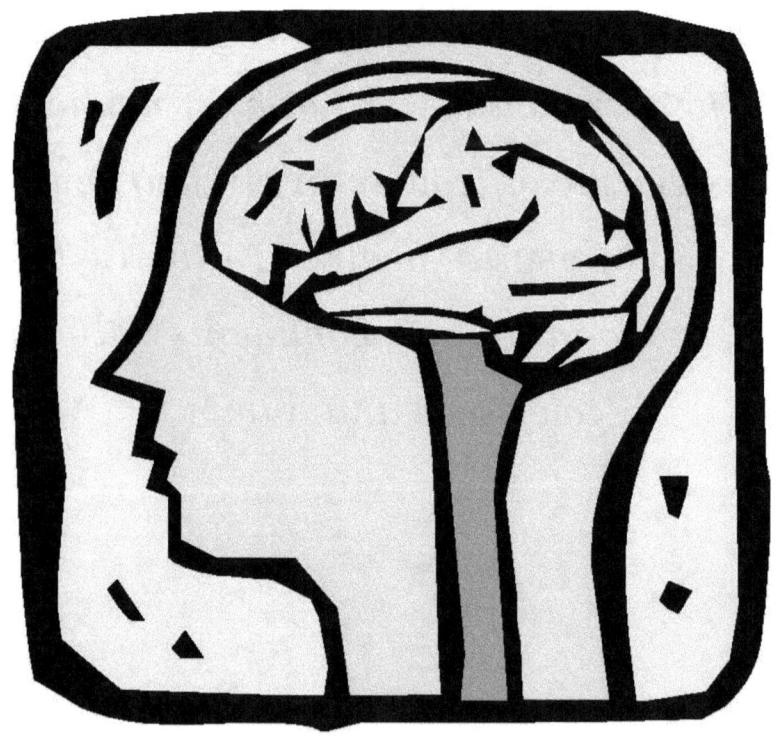

I believe people experience problems with depression and anxiety partly because of brain chemical dysregulation. Scientific data supports this belief. Medication helps me correct this chemical imbalance.

Reflections: _____

_____

_____

_____

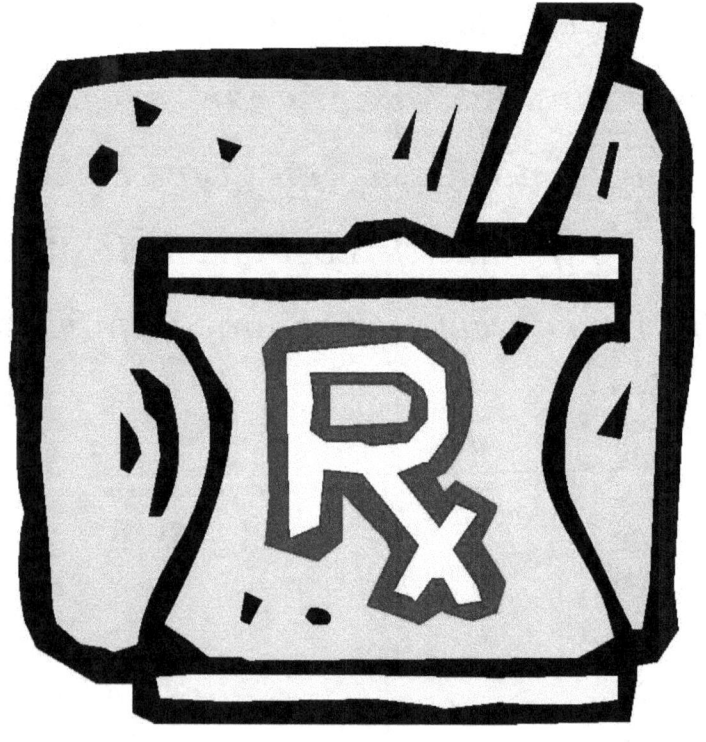

Some medications do not mix safely with other medications. Before I add any new medication, even over-the-counter medication, I will consult my clinician.

Reflections: _____

_____

_____

_____

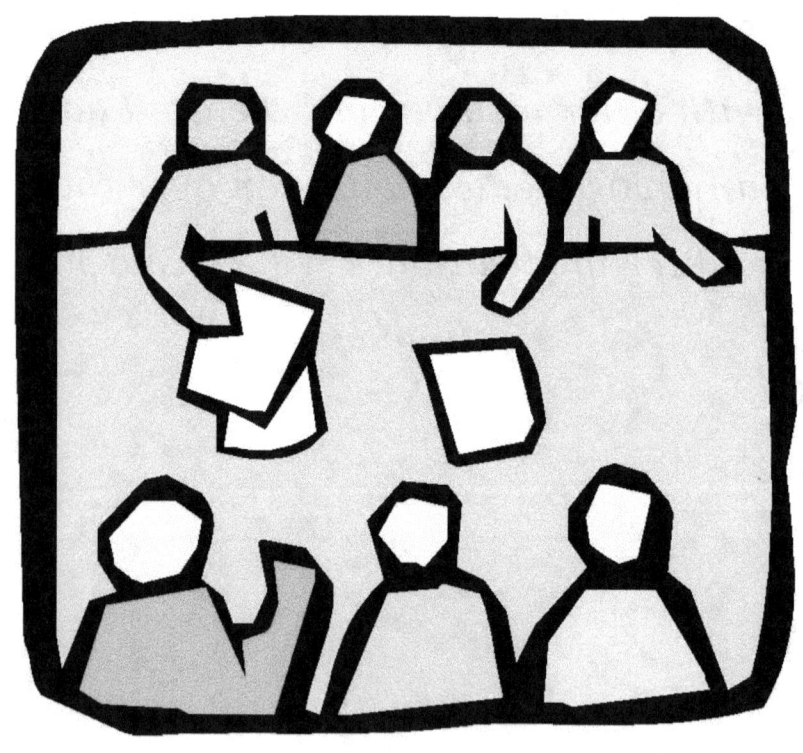

I am further empowered by joining support groups that are dedicated to serving the needs of people affected by depression and anxiety. In appropriate situations, I am an advocate for medication. Service to others furthers my healing.

Reflections: _____

_____

_____

_____

Mental Aerobics Project

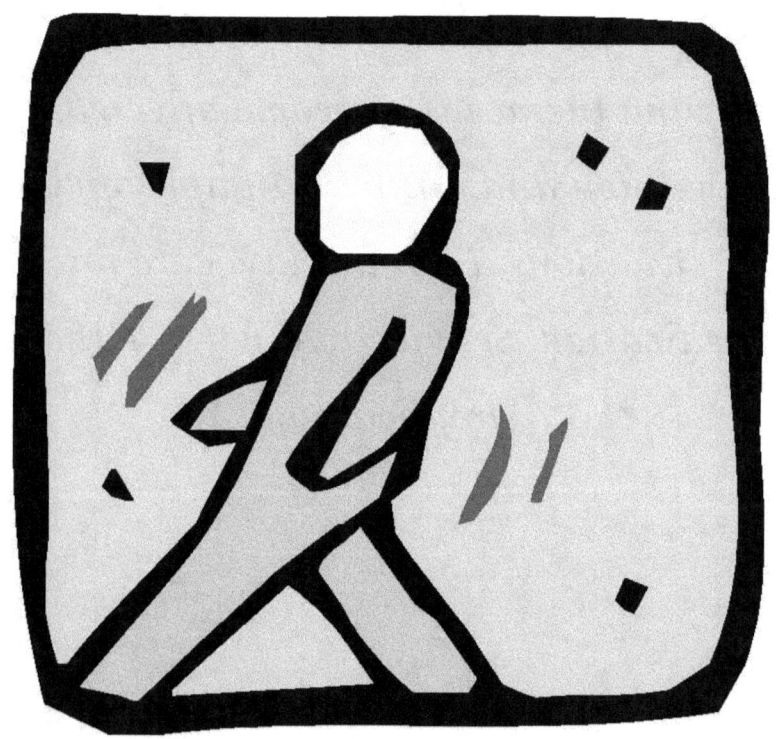

I gladly accept the benefits I receive from my medication. I will progress more quickly in therapy due to the reduction in depression and anxiety. I openly accept these benefits and continue to move forward with hope and anticipation.

Reflections: _____

_____

_____

_____

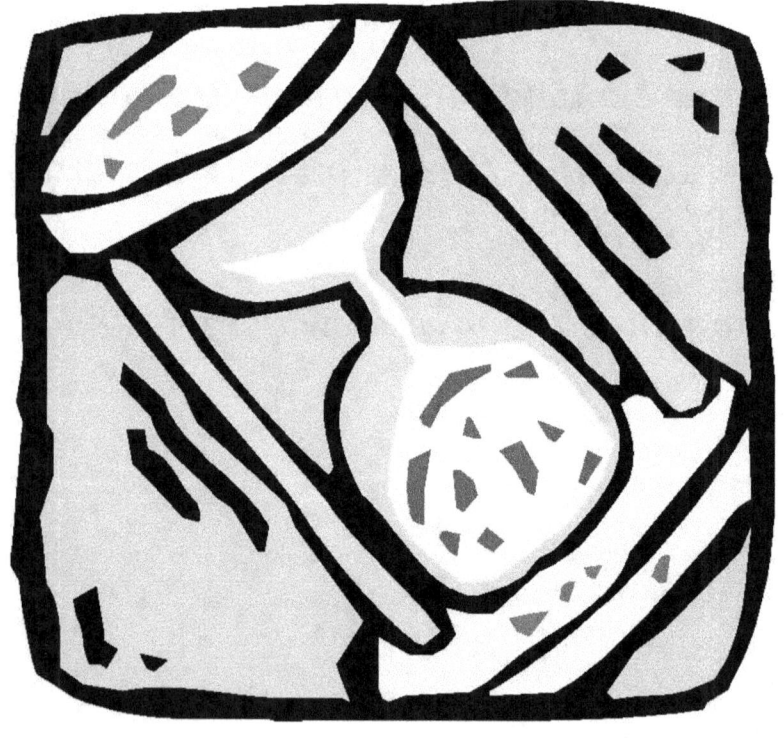

My patience is a virtue. It takes time to find the right medication and receive its full benefits.

Reflections: _____

_____

_____

_____

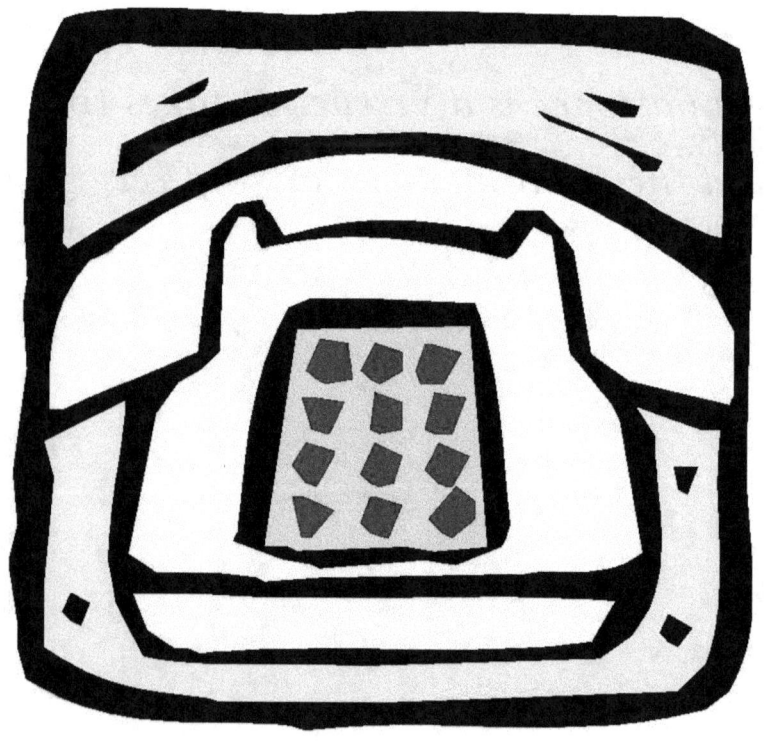

Taking medication for depression and anxiety is one way I choose to take care of myself. I will manage any thoughts of self-harm or suicide by immediately contacting my treatment team. I honor my life, cherish every moment, and relish each life-affirming breath.

Reflections: _____

_____

_____

_____

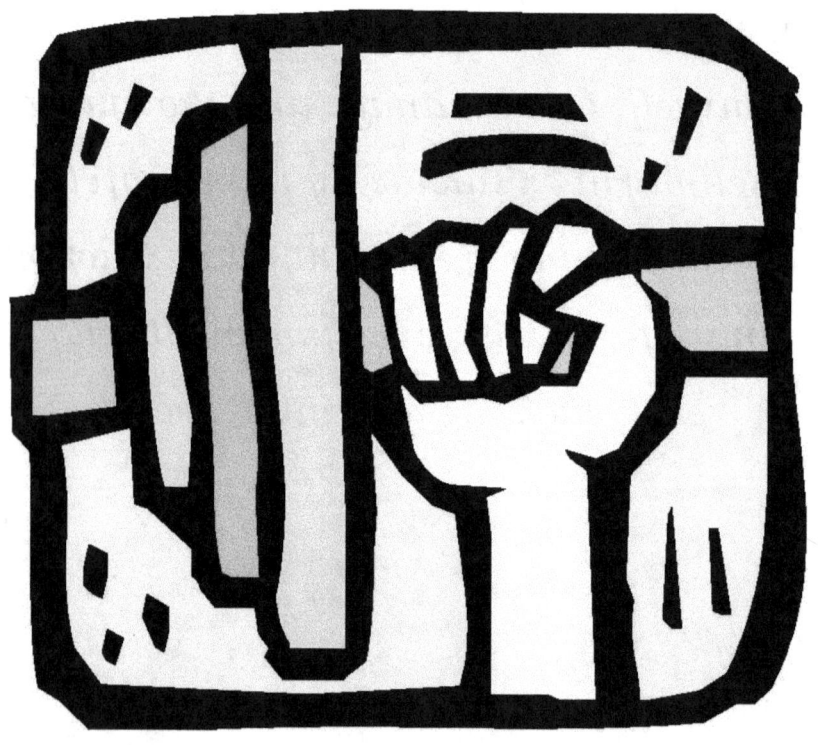

I honestly admit there are times I prefer not to take medication. My choice to take medication for depression and anxiety reflects my problem-solving attitude and wisdom. It is a sign of strength not weakness.

Reflections: _____

_____

_____

_____

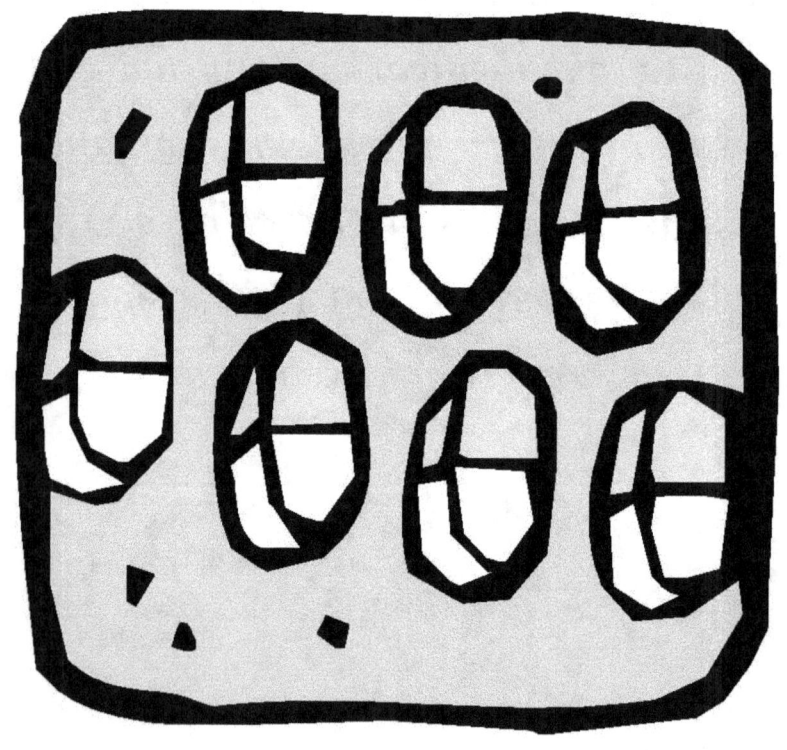

I accept the responsibilities associated with taking medication. I approach the duties of refilling prescriptions, calling my clinician, and actively participating in all aspects of my care with a positive attitude. I envision and embrace the outcome of health and happiness.

Reflections: _____

_____

_____

_____

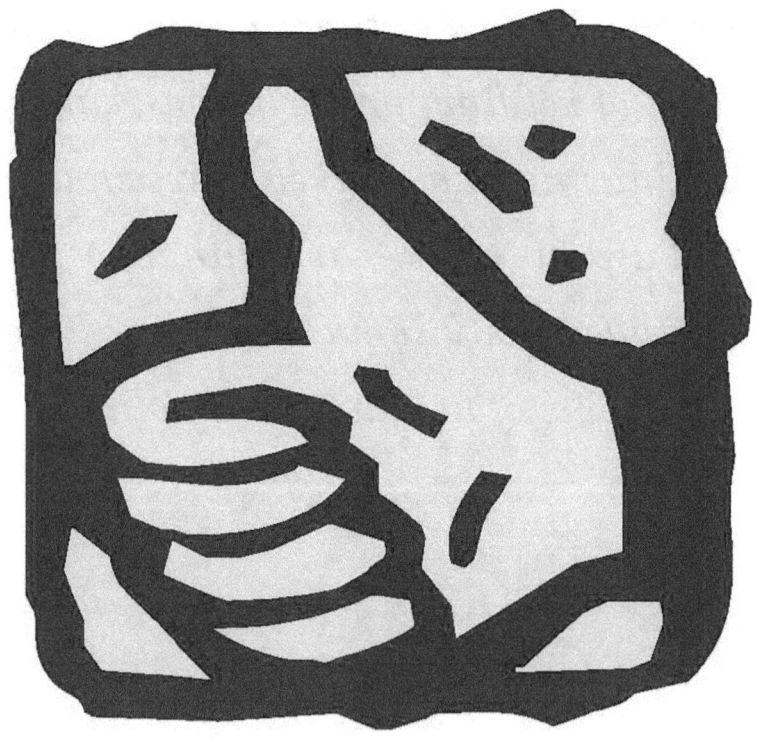

I believe in the power of my medication. This empowers me to change my life for the better.

Reflections: _____

_____

_____

_____

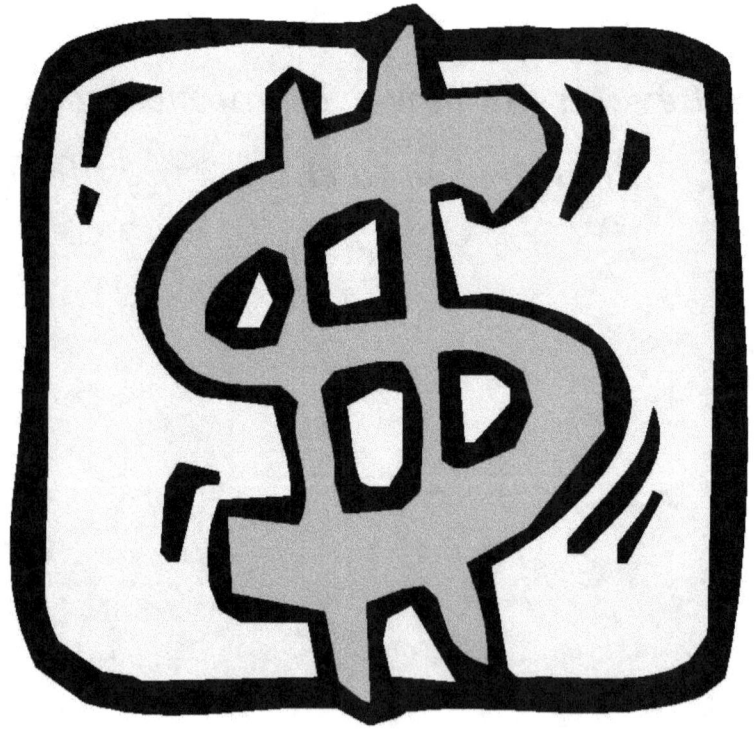

I may feel burdened by the financial stress of taking my medication. I will prioritize my needs and accomplish my goal of achieving good mental health. I am worth the investment.

Reflections: _____

_____

_____

_____

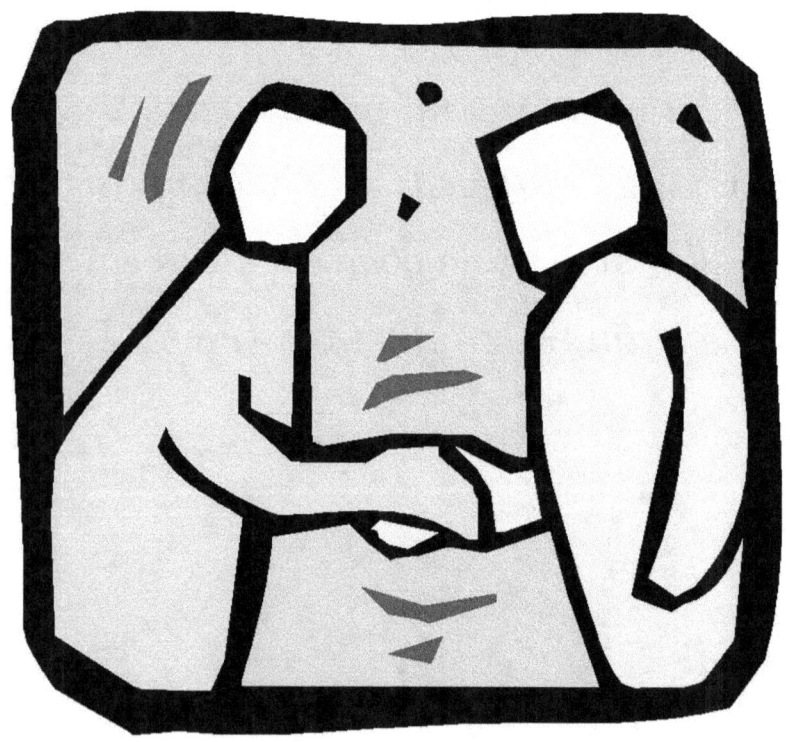

I am a positive person and believe in the power of partnership with my clinician. This healthy partnership will allow us to use the medication to its fullest.

Reflections: _____

_____

_____

_____

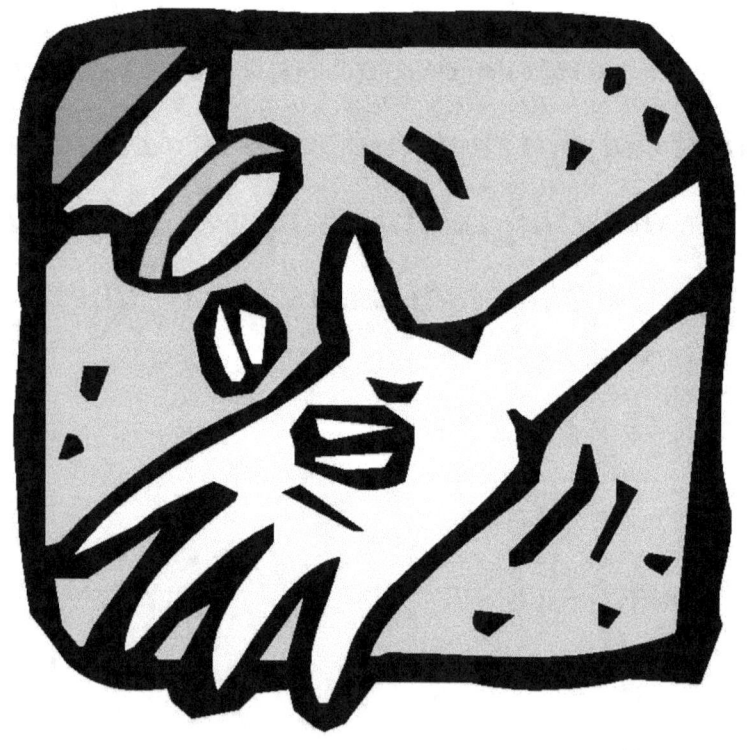

I respect all medications. I will take all medications responsibly.

Reflections: _____

_____

_____

_____

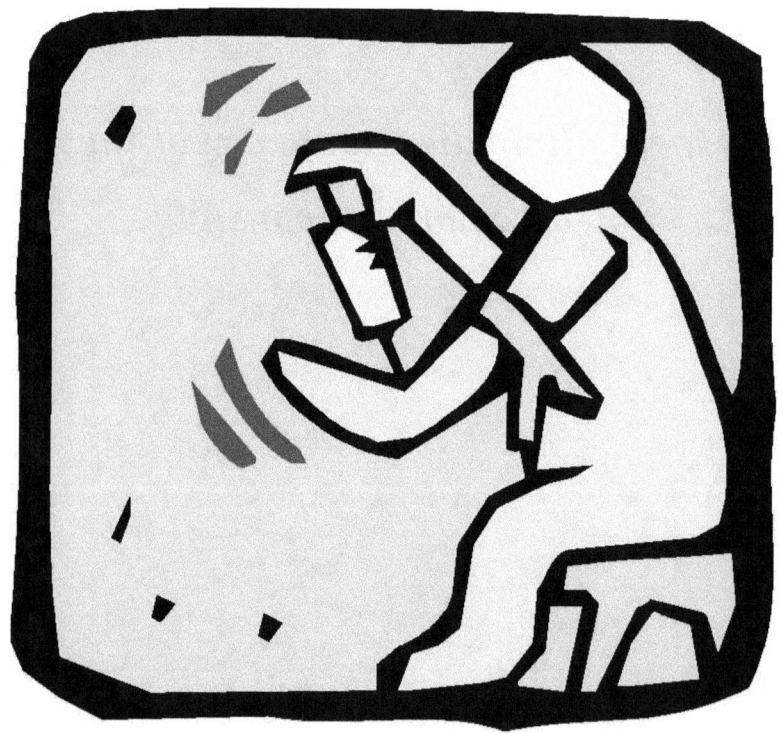

I am committed to leading a life free of addictions. I am aware all addictions are self-defeating behaviors. I will go forward with the help of my medication. I will not go backwards!

Reflections: _____

_____

_____

_____

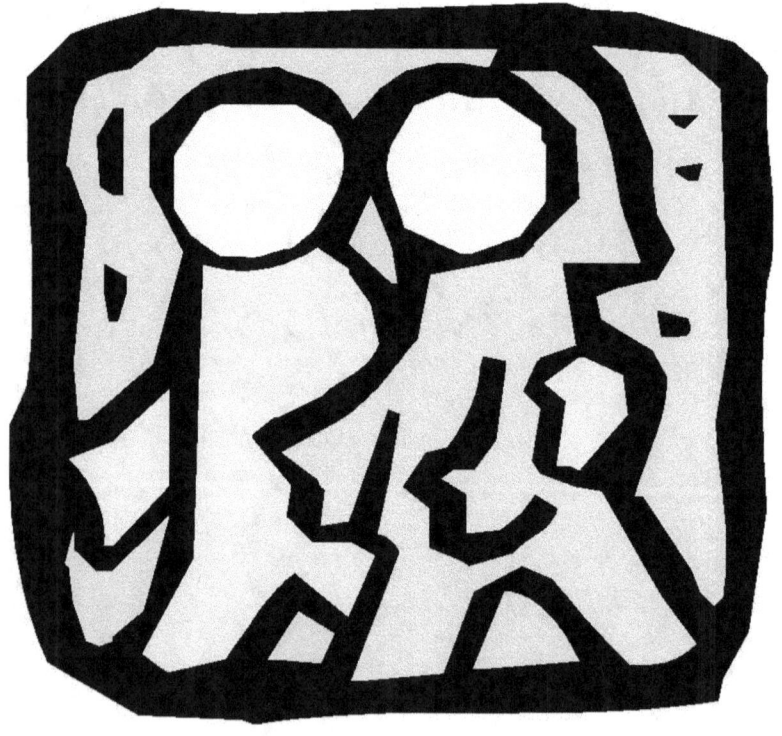

I am committed to friendships and socializing. I embrace the power to create and maintain friendships. Friendships are powerful aids in the fight against depression and anxiety. Utilizing this tool along with medication creates a strong defense. I feel empowered!

Reflections: _____

_____

_____

_____

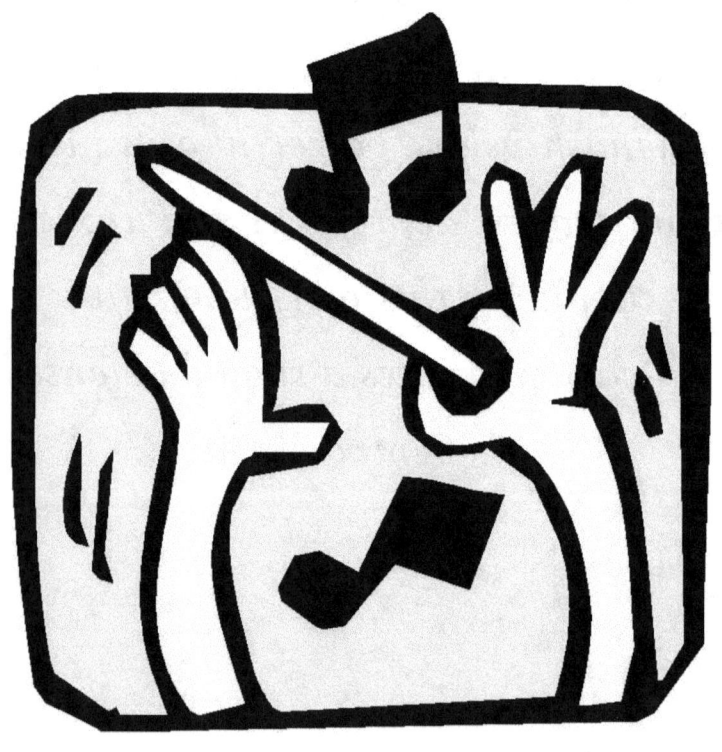

I will rely on each and every resource available to me: medication, exercise, good nutrition, therapy, spirituality, family, friends, work, mindfulness, and faith. As these work in harmony, I can achieve anything!

Reflections: _____

_____

_____

_____

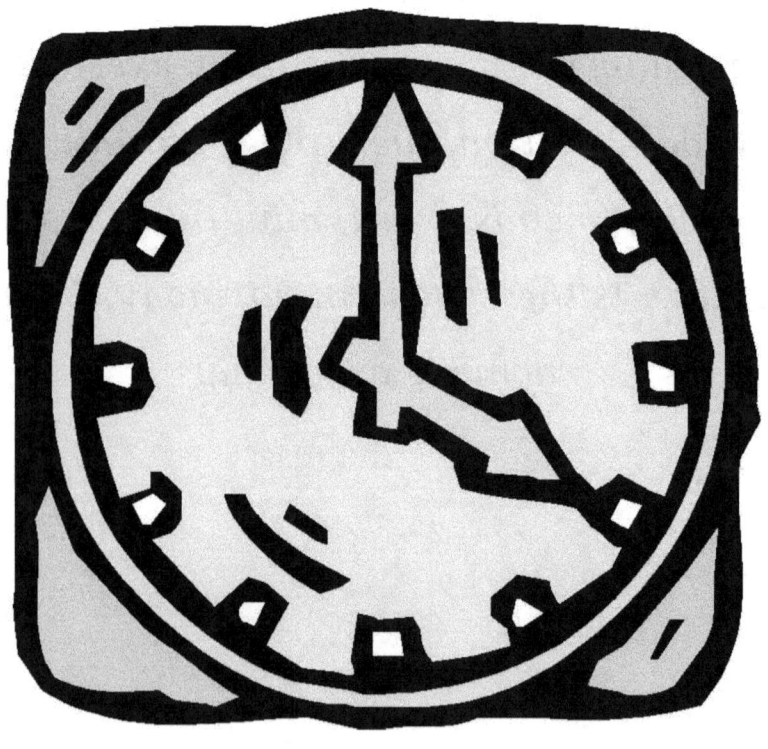

I accept the possibility of taking medication for an extended period of time if necessary. My knowledge has increased. I am a wiser person. If my clinician recommends long-term use of a medication, I will remain flexible and open-minded.

Reflections: _____

_____

_____

_____

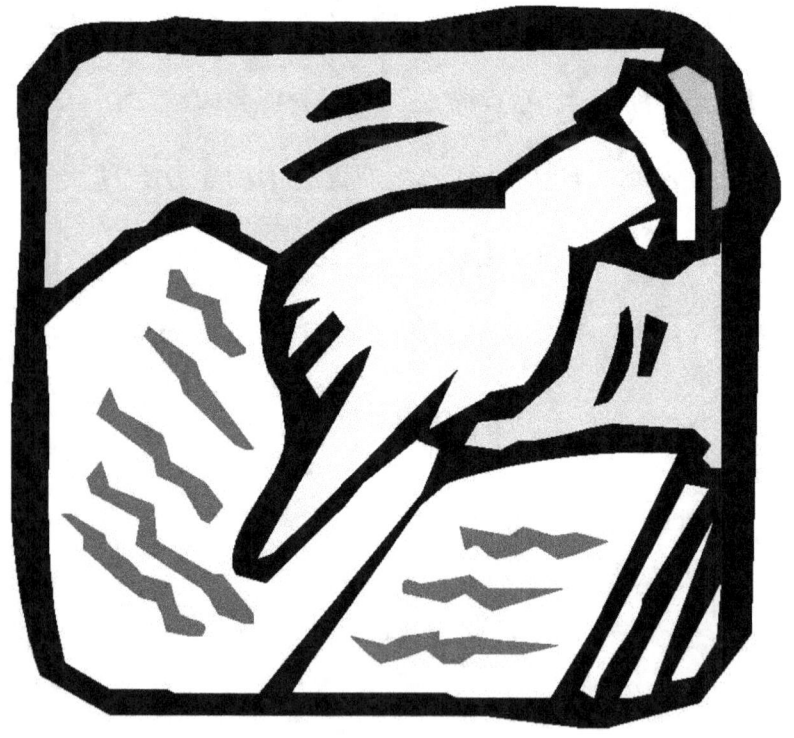

I am committed to education. I will teach my family and friends about mental health. I commit to helping others understand the role chemical imbalance plays in depression and anxiety. I will educate others about the benefits of medication. I will share my beliefs with others in a kind and gentle way.

Reflections: _____

_____

_____

_____

Mental Aerobics Project

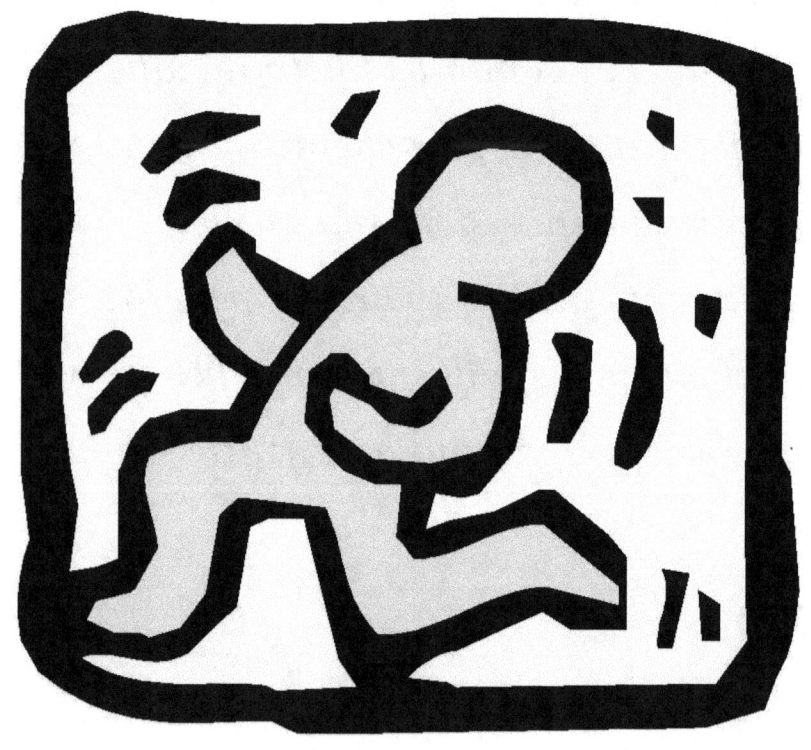

I commit to a physically active lifestyle. I will exercise daily. I will receive the full benefits of my medication as a result of this activity. So, I commit myself to get moving!!

Reflections: _____

_____

_____

_____

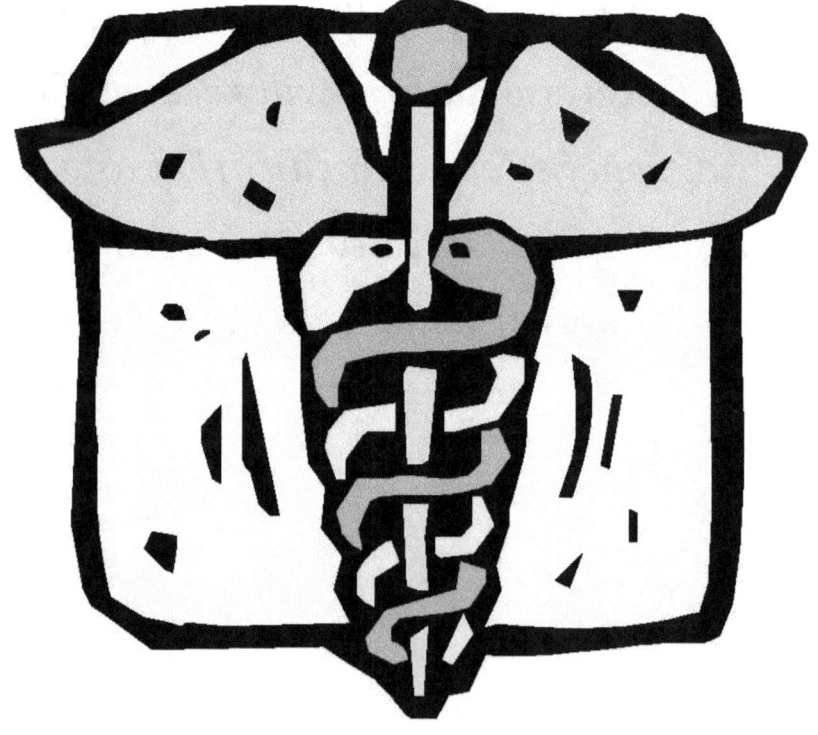

I believe depression and anxiety are medical illnesses, just like diabetes or any other physical illness. I view my medication the same way individuals with diabetes view insulin.

Reflections: _____

_____

_____

_____

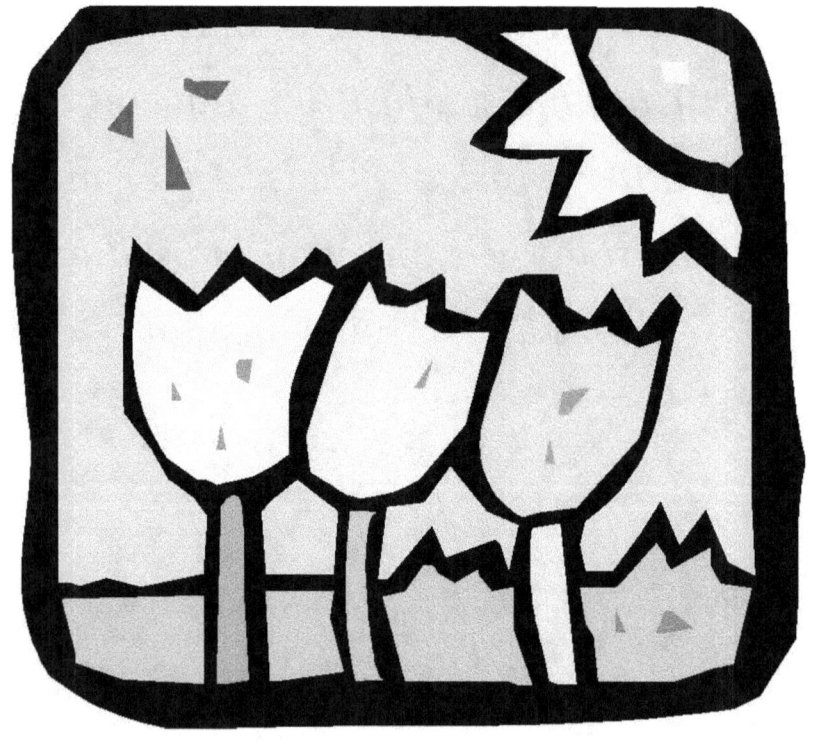

I will no longer criticize myself for needing medication. From today forward I accept this belief: "I choose to take medication so I can lead the best possible life. I honor my life and my ability to make good and sound decisions."

Reflections: _____

_____

_____

_____

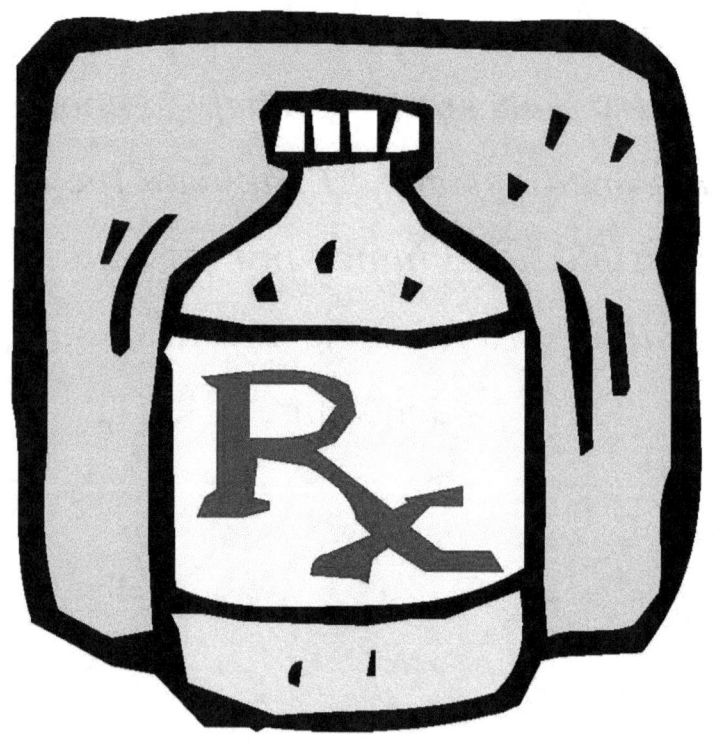

I promise to take my medication regularly and as prescribed. To not do so is to cheat myself. I am dedicated to taking great care of myself ---- forever!

Reflections: _____

_____

_____

_____

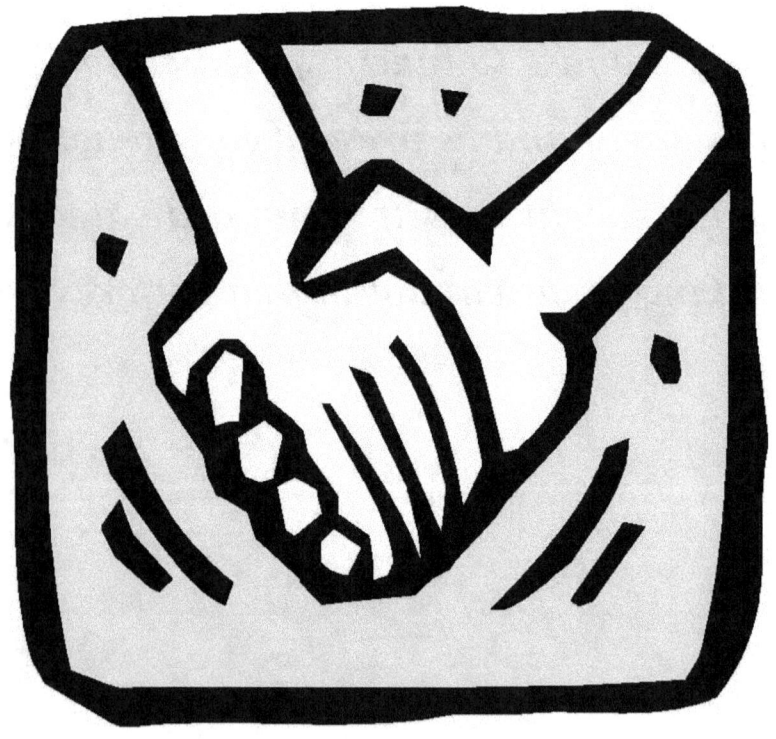

I will view medication in a kinder and more compassionate way. Anger, distrust, disrespect, and rejection play no role in my relationship with medication. I commit to developing a productive and beneficial relationship with my medication.

Reflections: _____

_____

_____

_____

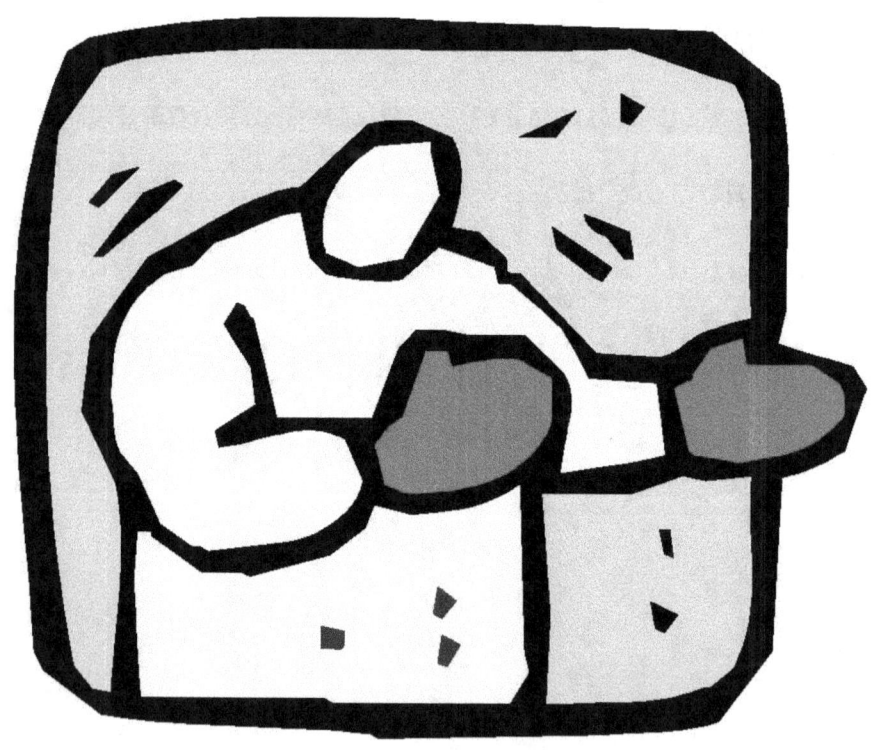

I am a fighter not a victim! Medication is one of the powerful weapons in my fight against depression and anxiety.

Reflections: _____

_____

_____

_____

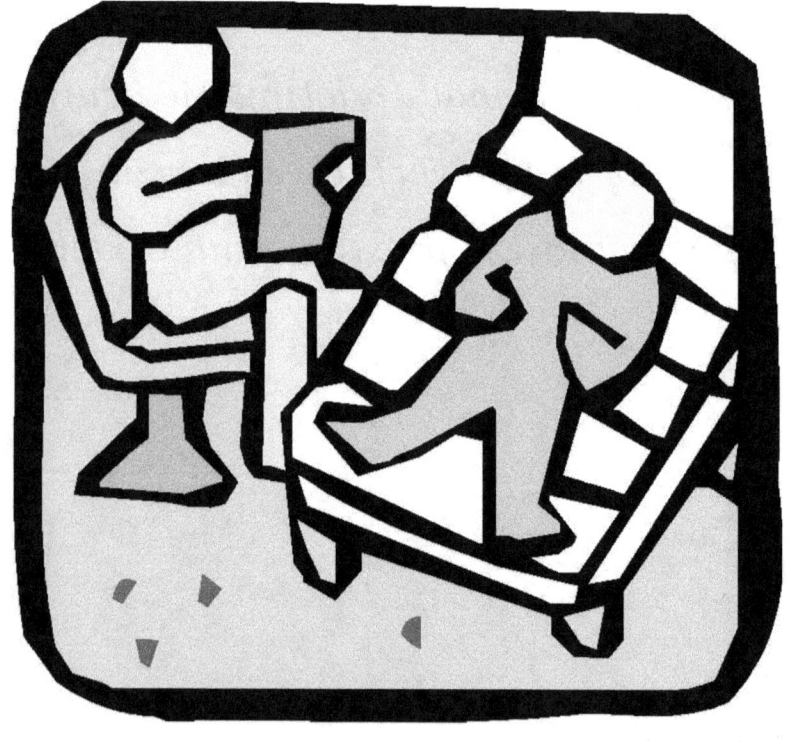

I am committed to search for a competent and compassionate clinician. To truly benefit from medication and therapy I must feel listened to and cared for. I deserve only the best!

Reflections: _____

_____

_____

_____

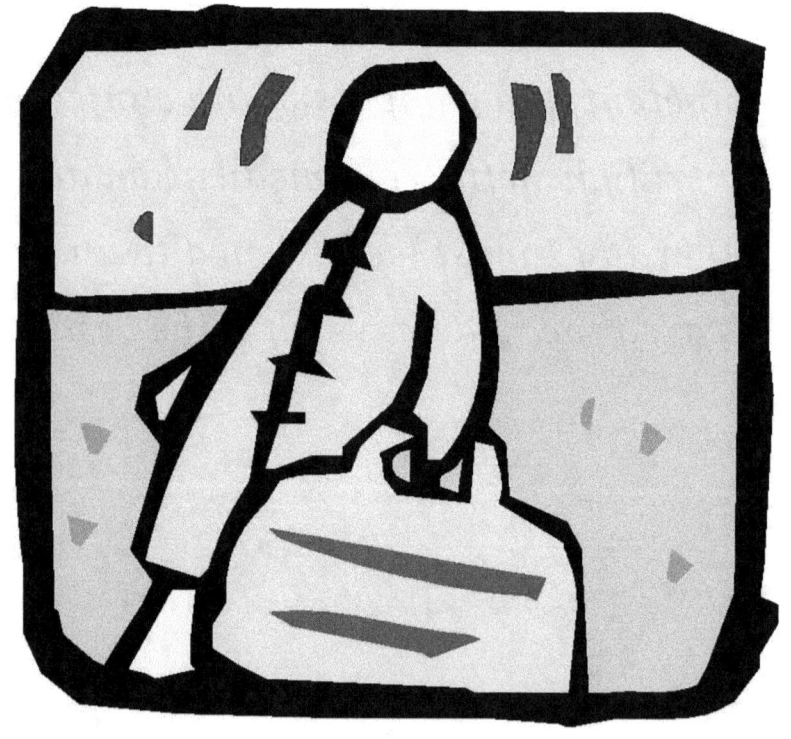

I choose to take care of my mental health and enlist the help of medication. Achieving the fullest potential is my goal. Medication supports my journey.

Reflections: _____

_____

_____

_____

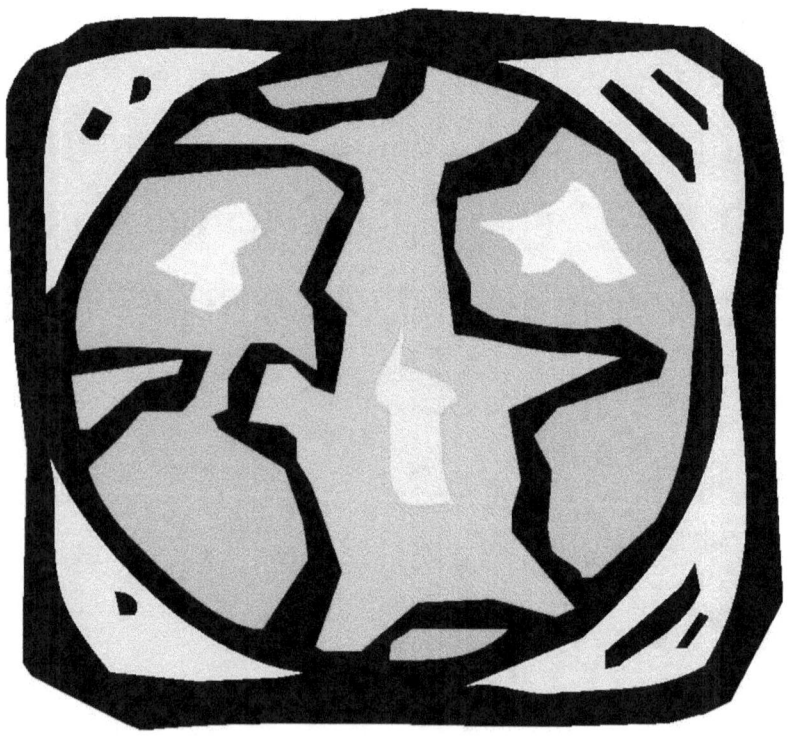

I know the world is not a perfect place. Even on medication my symptoms of depression and anxiety may resurface. I am not frightened by this possibility. I choose to maintain a calm watch over my moods and anxiety. I will keep my clinician informed of any problems.

Reflections: _____

_____

_____

_____

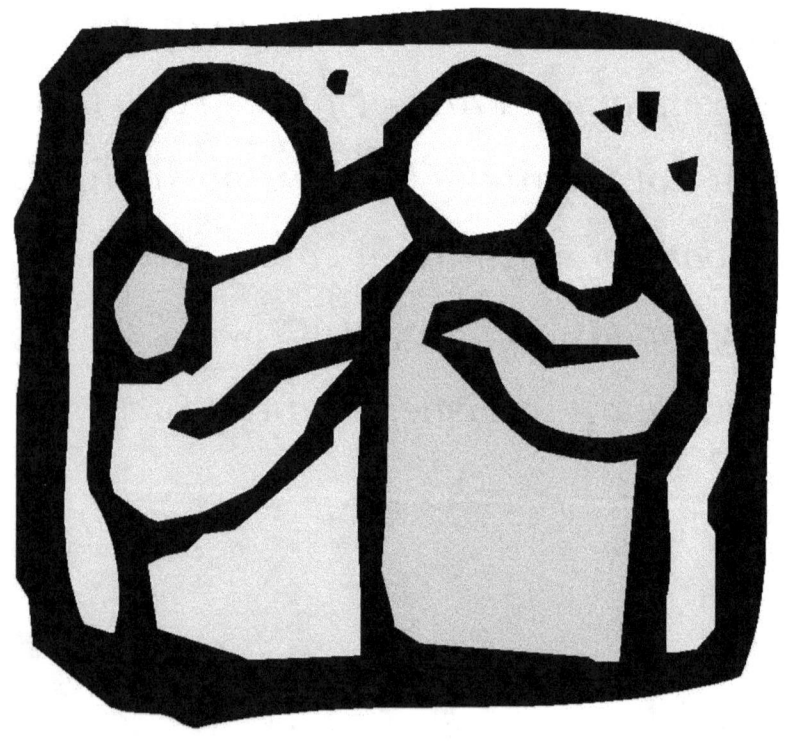

The relationship I have with my medication is like a friendship. Conflict plays a role in all friendships. I will learn to peacefully and respectfully resolve all conflicts. This friendship is one of joy, growth, and prosperity.

Reflections: _____

_____

_____

_____

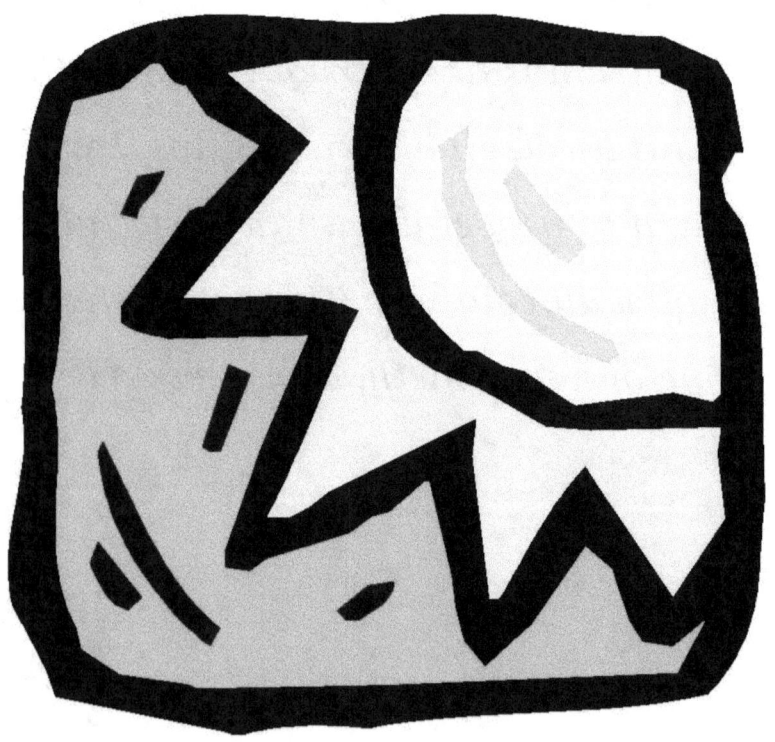

I do not accept feelings of shame because I take medication. I am nourishing my mind, body, and spirit in a journey toward health and wellness. Shame plays no part in this adventure.

Reflections: _____

_____

_____

_____

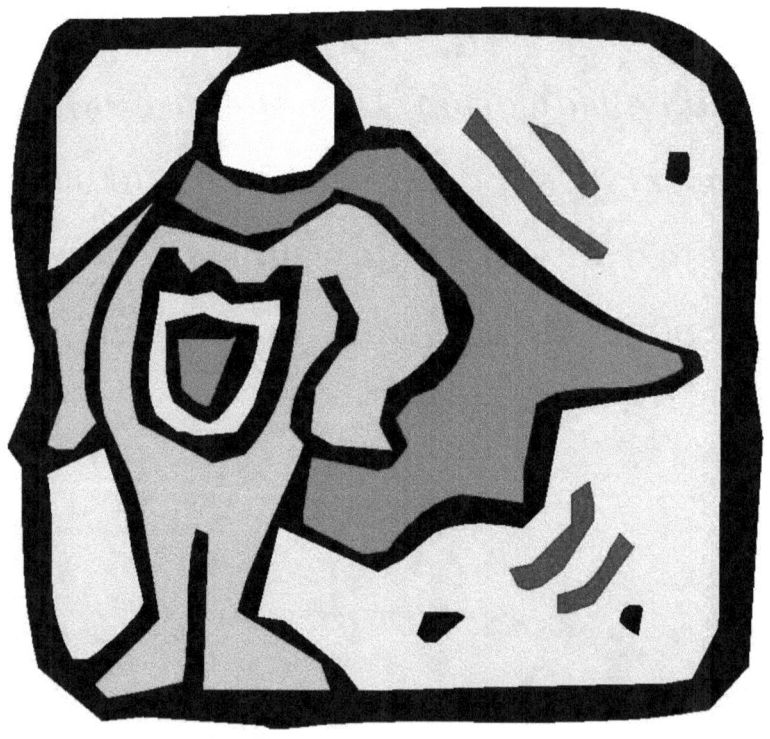

I am a role model for others dealing with the negative effects of depression and anxiety. I offer my guidance, support, and help to others interested in making positive changes.

Reflections: _____

_____

_____

_____

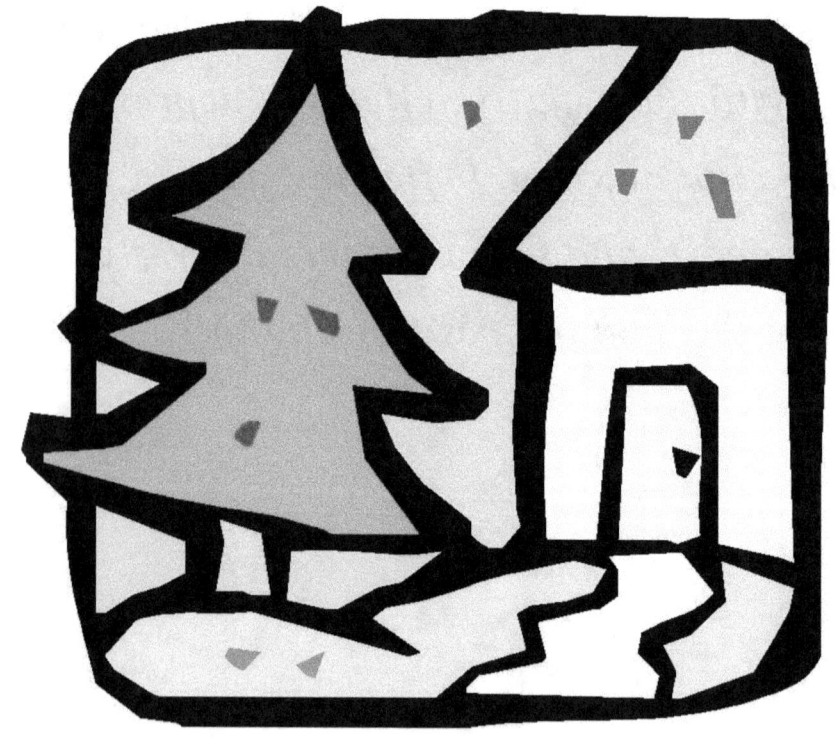

I will store my medication in a safe and secure place. No one, not even my pets, will have access to my medication. My home is safe for all those that enter.

Reflections: _____

_____

_____

_____

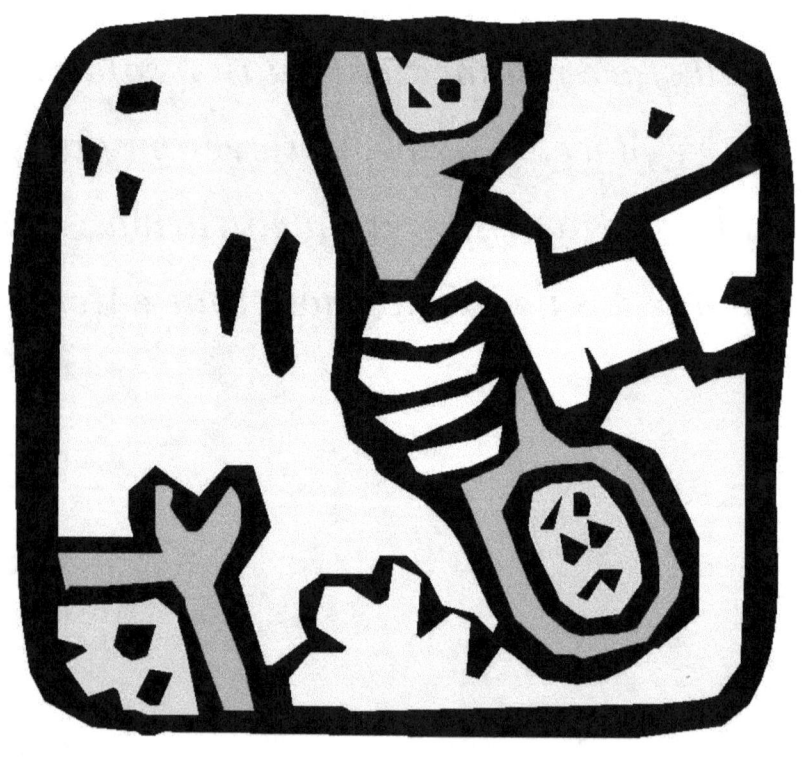

I commit to open communication with my clinician. I am watchful for possible medication side effects. If they occur, I will report them to my clinician immediately. Possible side effects might include sleep and weight changes, sexual life changes, nausea, headaches, etc.

Reflections: _____

_____

_____

_____

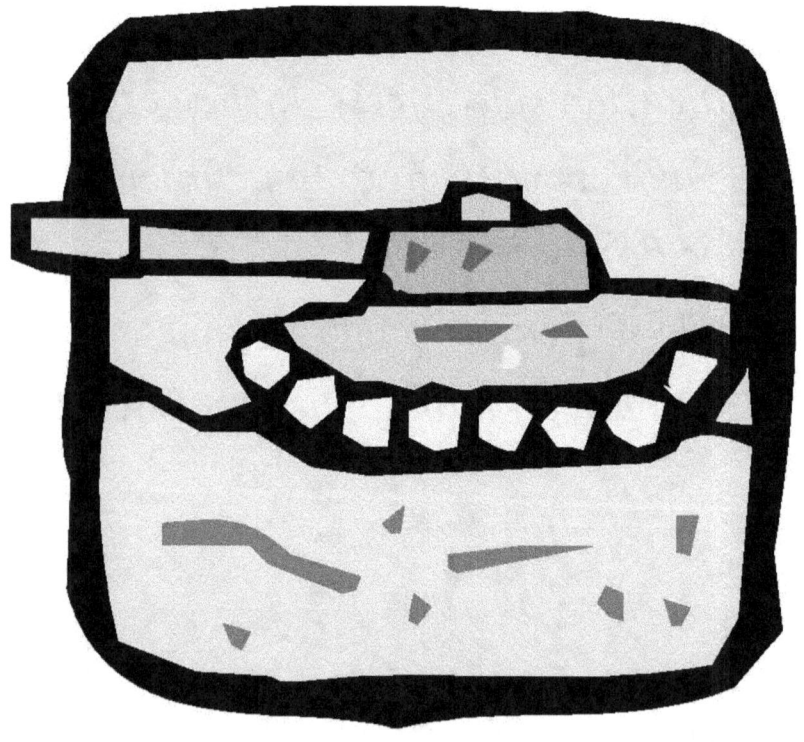

I recognize the destructive power of depression and anxiety. I am committed to doing all I can to harness this destructive force. Medication is one weapon I choose to use in my battle against depression and anxiety.

Reflections: _____

_____

_____

_____

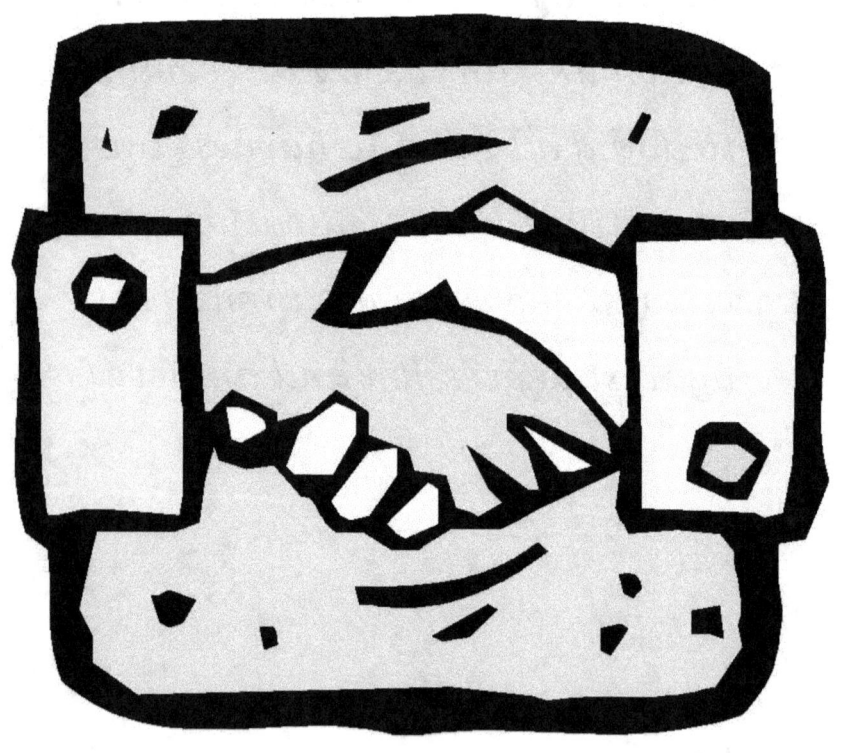

I know medication may cause side effects. I am committed to telling my clinician about any problems I encounter. I benefit from the powerful partnership we share.

Reflections: _____

_____

_____

_____

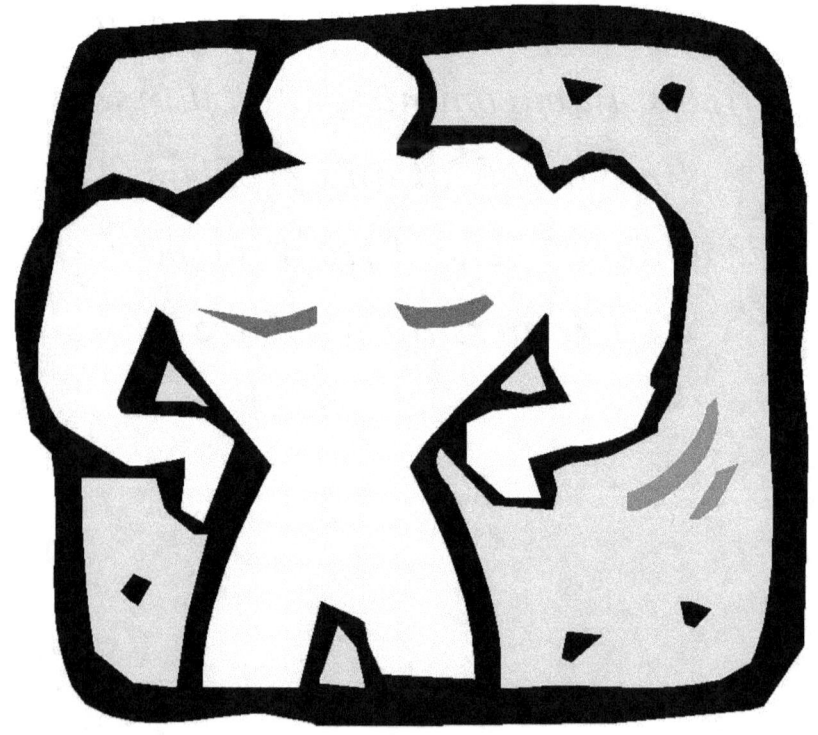

Medication makes me stronger in my ability to manage my depression and anxiety.

Reflections: _____

_____

_____

_____

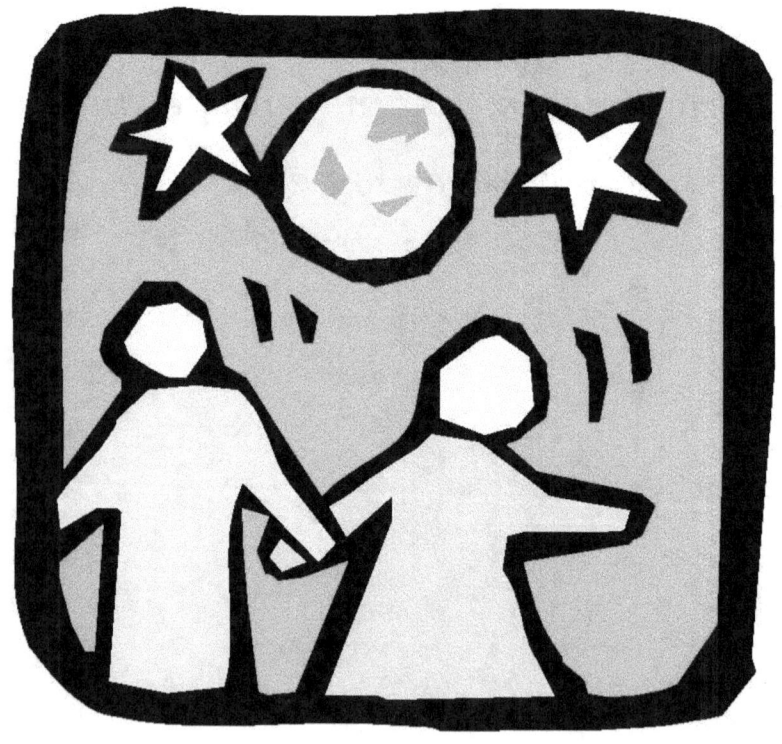

I commit to a balanced lifestyle. Medication helps me achieve this goal. I embrace the help of positive thoughts, positive actions, and positive relationships in my life.

Reflections: _____

_____

_____

_____

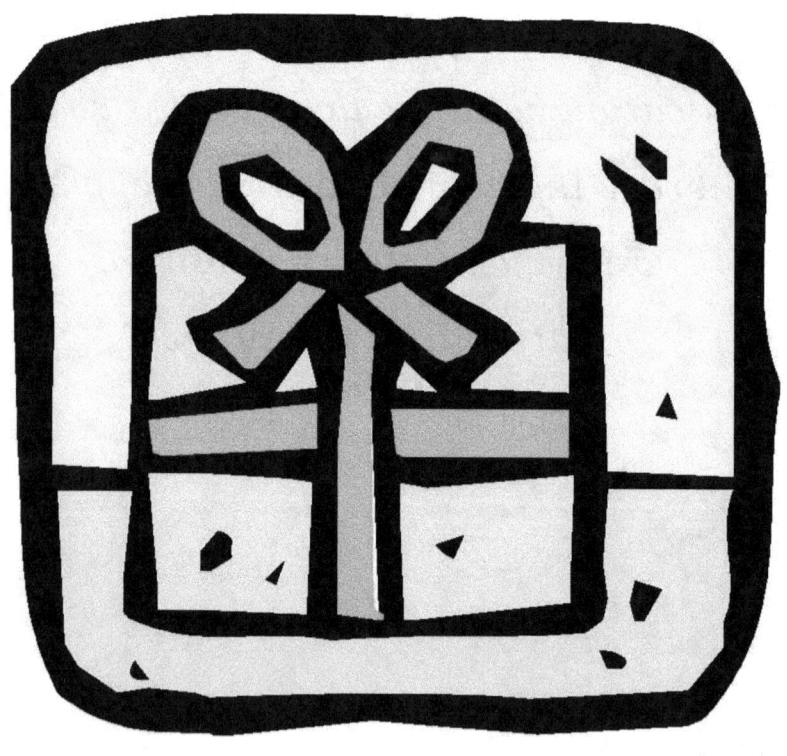

God's gifts are plentiful and abundant. Medication to control my depression and anxiety is one such gift. I freely accept the gift with gratitude and love.

Reflections: _____

_____

_____

_____

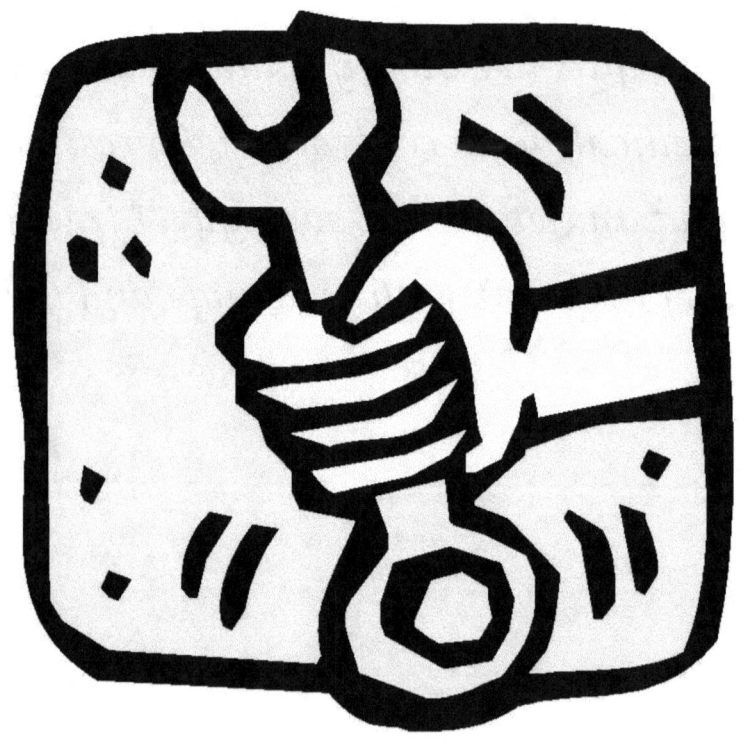

I recognize even the best of tools have limitations. I am committed to doing all I can to ensure my medications are successful. I remain positive and strong in my journey.

Reflections: _____

_____

_____

_____

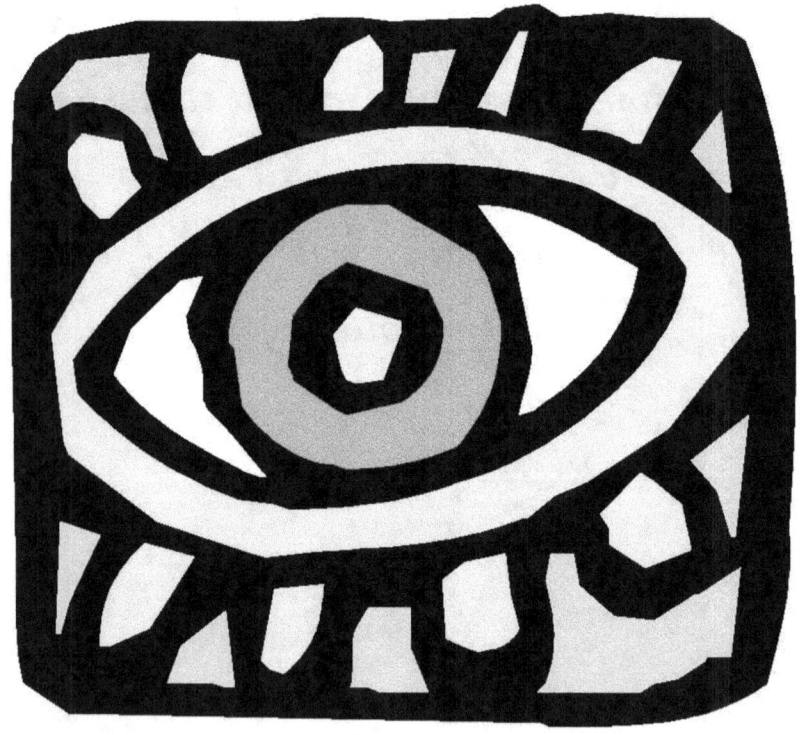

I promise to work cooperatively with my clinician. If we agree to a trial of stopping my medication, I will proceed slowly and remain watchful for signs of depression and anxiety. I will follow my clinician's directions. My goal is to protect myself in all endeavors.

Reflections: _____

_____

_____

_____

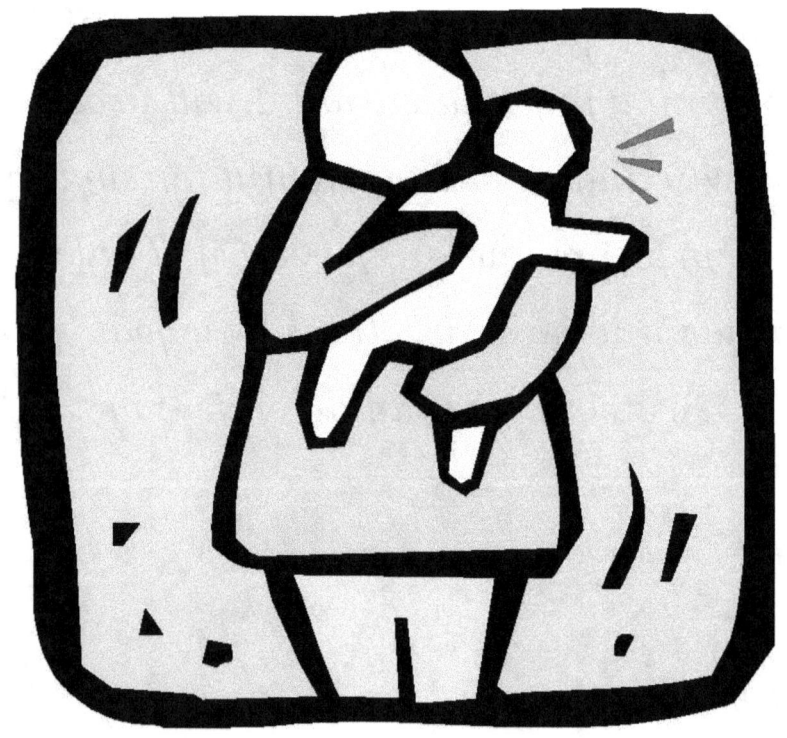

The decision to have a child demands thoughtful attention, especially while taking medication. I agree to discuss this option with my clinician prior to making a decision. I am committed to the journey of health, growth, and prosperity.

Reflections: _____

_____

_____

_____

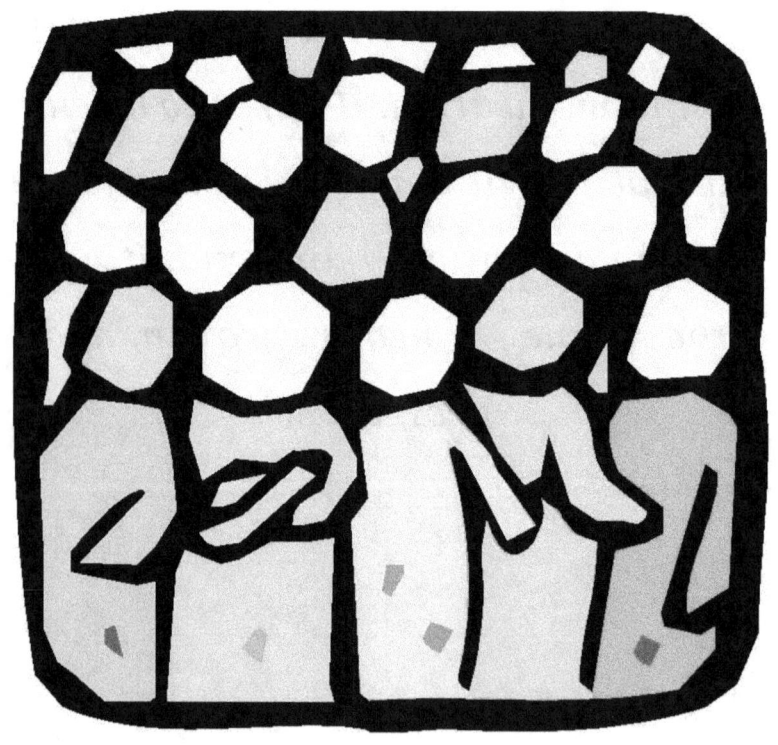

I acknowledge the benefits I receive from taking medication. Everyone in my life shares in the benefits.

Reflections: _____

_____

_____

_____

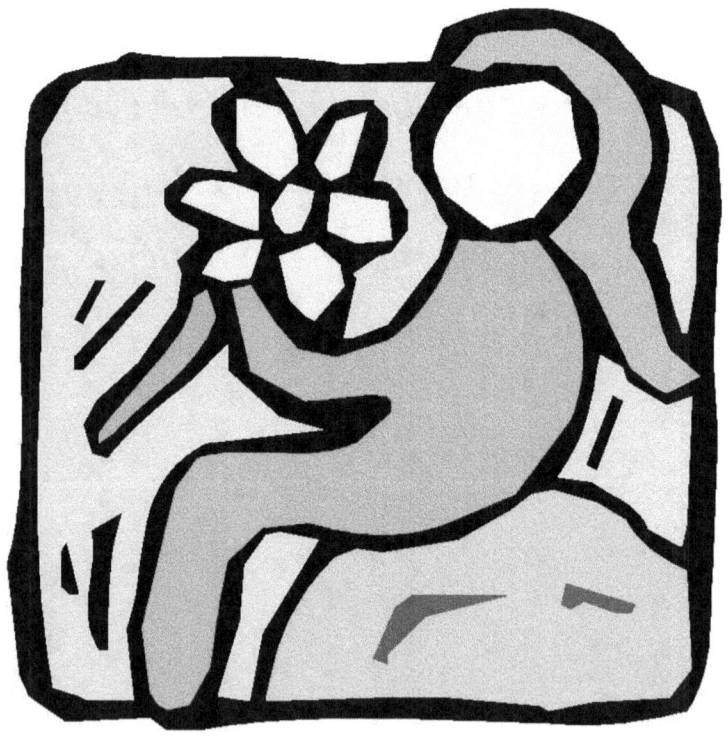

I am not defined by the medication I choose to take. To the contrary, wisdom, courage, and strength to make the right decisions to improve my life define me.

Reflections: _____

_____

_____

_____

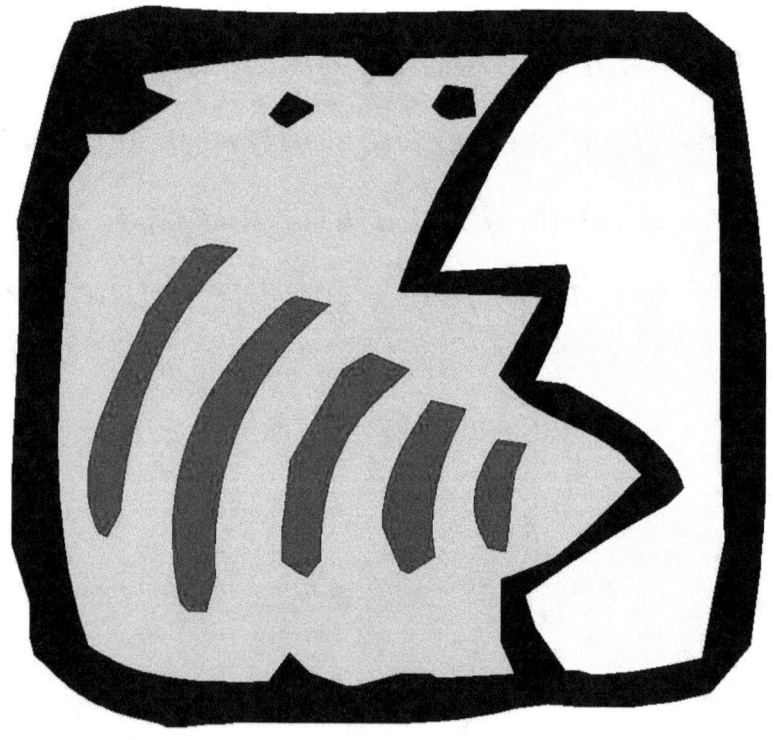

I will not stop taking my medication without consulting my clinician. I am fully committed to my mental health and well being. I will talk to my clinician before making any decisions about my medication.

Reflections: _____

_____

_____

_____

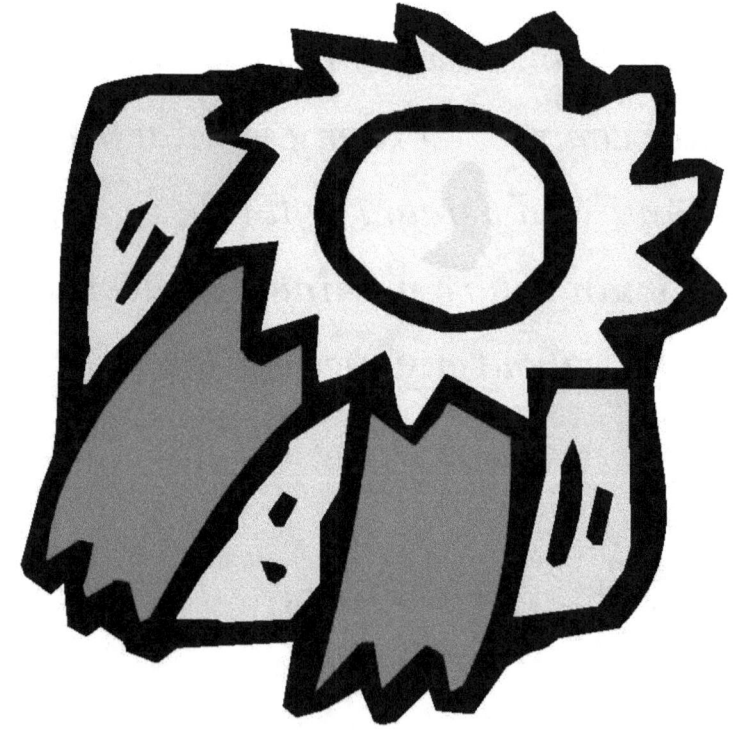

I do not choose to suffer from depression and anxiety. I am responsible for controlling the negative effect it has on my life and my family. My choice to take medication is one way I can win over depression and anxiety.

Reflections: _____

_____

_____

_____

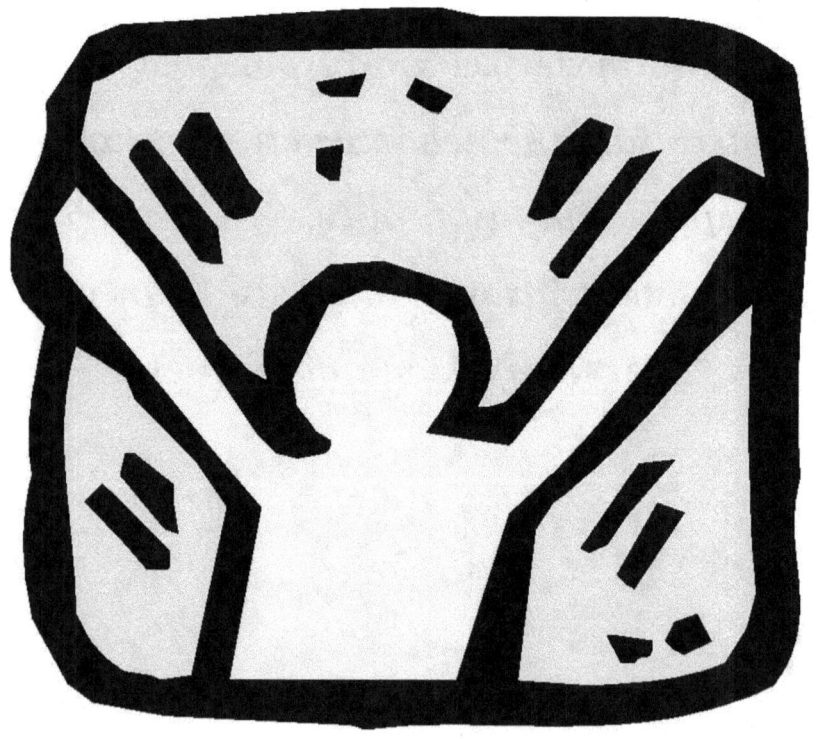

I commit to conquering depression and anxiety for the rest of my life. I will take advantage of all the tools available to me and continue to search for new ones. Medication is one of the tools available to me. I am blessed to have access to this powerful tool.

Reflections: _____

_____

_____

_____

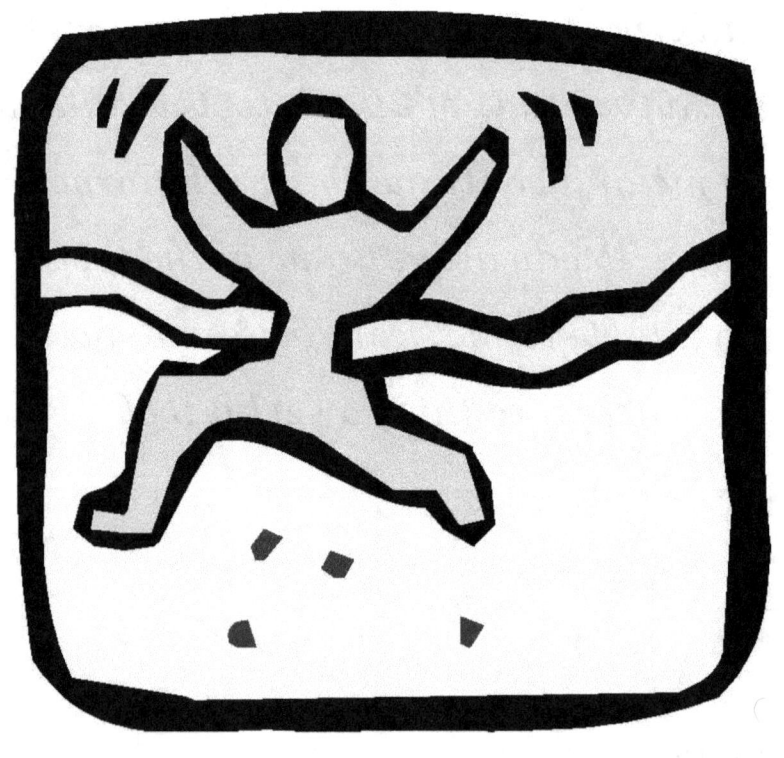

I have depression and anxiety.

Depression and anxiety do not have me!

Reflections: _____

_____

_____

_____

ABOUT THE AUTHORS

Saundra Jain, MA, PsyD, LPC is the Executive Director of the *Mental Aerobics Project* (MAP). MAP is focused on wellness and the impact of positive psychology on patient outcomes. Dr. Jain provides workshops to both healthcare practitioners, organizations, businesses and individuals interested in learning more about the power of wellness. In 1992, she launched a private practice of psychotherapy where she currently provides services for a wide range of mental health issues.

Dr. Jain is very active in the area of peer–to–peer education especially in the disease states of depression, bipolar disorder, and ADHD. Another strong clinical and educational interest involves differential diagnosis of major psychiatric disorders. She is the co–creator and co–presenter of a novel and extremely well received interactive workshop/program addressing the challenges of dealing with psychiatric co–morbidities through the use of psychiatric scales and screeners. This program reached a national audience and, according to many attendees, changed the way they practice medicine. She has been instrumental in developing several other innovative tools/programs to fill current gaps in this area. She is the co–creator and co–presenter featured on an interactive DVD titled *"Differentiating Bipolar Depression from Unipolar Depression"*. Recently, Dr. Jain served as the co–host of *"Depression in Relationships"* a medical education program broadcasted in 20 major cities in the United States on several major television networks (NBC, ABC, CBS and FOX) and the Voice of America national news & talk radio system.

She obtained her Masters degree from the University of Houston-Clear Lake and a Doctoral degree from California Southern University for Professional Studies. She demonstrated her professional versatility by obtaining an MBA from Texas Woman's University. She is a Licensed Professional Counselor and member of the American Association for Marriage and Family Therapy. She has extensive clinical training in multiple sites, covering the gamut of childhood, adolescent and adult experiences in both the private and the public sector. She was selected for a Postgraduate

Clinical Fellowship at the University of Texas Medical Branch, Galveston, Texas where she trained in the Division of Child and Adolescent Psychiatry.

Rakesh Jain, MD, MPH is Associate Clinical Professor of Psychiatry, University of Texas Medical School in Houston, Texas and Director of Psychiatric Drug Research for the R/D Clinical Research Center in Lake Jackson, Texas.

Dr. Jain attended medical school at the University of Calcutta in India. He then attended graduate school at the University of Texas School of Public Health in Houston, where he was awarded a National Institute/Center for Disease Control Competitive Traineeship. His research thesis focused on the impact of substance abuse. He graduated from the School of Public Health in 1987 with a Masters of Public Health (MPH) degree.

After graduate school, Dr. Jain completed a postdoctoral fellowship in Research Psychiatry at the University of Texas Mental Sciences Institute in Houston. He received the National Research Service Award for the support of the postdoctoral fellowship. After this, he served a three-year residency in Psychiatry at the Department of Psychiatry and Behavioral Sciences at the University of Texas Medical School at Houston as well as a two-year fellowship in Child and Adolescent Psychiatry.

Dr. Jain is currently involved in multiple research projects studying the effects of medications on short-term and long-term treatment of depression, anxiety, pain/mood overlap disorders, and psychosis in adult and child/adolescent populations. He is the author of several articles on the issue of mood and pain conditions. His research posters have been presented at the APA, ACNP, AACAP, US Psychiatric Congress, among others. He has been a co-author on several articles written for peer-reviewed journals such as *Journal of Psychiatric Research*, *Journal of Clinical Psychiatry*, among others. He has presented recently at the World Psychiatric Congress held in Prague, and at the Pain Forum meetings in Greece, Brazil, Portugal, United Kingdom, and Argentina.

He serves on several Advisory Boards focusing on drug development and disease state education. He was recently named "Public Citizen of the Year" by the National Association of Social Workers, Gulf Coast Chapter, in recognition of community and peer education and championing of mental health issues. He was also awarded the "Extra Mile Award" by Brazosport Independent School District, in recognition of his service to the children of the school district and consultation to the teachers and counselors. In 2008, at the U.S. Psychiatric Congress, held in San Diego, California, he was the recipient of "Teacher of the Year Award." He was also the Chair of the Steering Committee for the 2009 US Psychiatric Congress, held in Las Vegas in November 2009 and currently serves on its Steering Committee.

The authors are available for workshops,
seminars, and speaking engagements.
For more details, visit their web site at
www.mentalaerobicsproject.com.